BLOOD WOR
INTERPRETA
MANUAL

**The Ultimate Guide to
Understanding How to Read
Blood Test and Interpret
Blood Work to Improve
Quality of Life and Wellness**

June Corder

1

TABLE OF CONTENT

CHAPTER 1

INTRODUCTION

First let's speak about why the results of blood tests are so essential. It is useful to consider your blood as both an oxygen supply system and a waste disposal process.

Some of your body's organs, including your liver, kidneys, spleen and lungs, function as processing points. Standard values imply healthy organ function and fully operating systems in a lab result.

Normal areas are defined by testing a large number of healthy people. It is crucial to remember that out-of-range test findings are not necessarily an indication of an oncoming disease.

However, a variety of variables, including age, sex, weight, medical history, medications and lifestyles, might alter these ranges. Your doctor will best assess what is "normal" for you.

CHAPTER 2

BLOOD TESTS AND HOW TO READ THEM

Below is a useful way to decode a blood test sample.

Learn to read the results of your wellness blood tests!

1. The BUN urea nitrogen test is used to examine the function of the kidney. The test measures your urine's urea or nitrogen levels.

In general, normal BUN levels vary between 6 to 20 (mg/dL) in people.

Higher levels of BUN may include dehydration, renal failure or illness, excessive protein levels, heart failure, gastrointestinal hemorrhage, or urinary tract blockage.

Lower BUN levels might suggest insufficient liver, malnutrition or a severe protein shortage in your diet.

So if you have a number over 21, investigate the likelihood of the first group of illnesses with your doctor. And, if it is under 6, the second group of illnesses should be checked.

2. The total protein test examines the amount of albumin and globulin in your body.

Understanding your protein blood test results... The typical range is between 6 and 8.3 (g/dL) for the total protein.

High protein can lead to inflammation or infections, such viral hepatitis B, viral hepatitis C or HIV. It can also indicate abnormalities of the bone marrow.

Blooding, liver disorders, renal problem, malnutrition or inflammatory conditions might suggest low protein.

Bet you didn't even consider you may have greater or lower protein levels. Now, if you don't receive enough or have too much, you know what it implies.

3. The sodium serum test measures your blood sodium.

The typical sodium range is 136-145 (mmol/L).

High sodium might imply your diet is dehydrated and you don't drink enough water and eat too much sodium. The symptoms of low sodium under active surrender glands, kidney failure, heart failure or thyroid gland might be low sodium.

Sweating, burning, diarrhea or poor diet may also induce low sodium.

So much sodium is concealed in food. It's very simple to overdo!

4. Total cholesterol test evaluates your blood's level of waxy fat-like cholesterol. Both LDL (bad) and HDL (good) cholesterol will be examined in the cholesterol total test.

The normal cholesterol range is lower than 200 (mg/dL).

Total high cholesterol is 240 (mg/dL), higher and dangerous.

And borderline high risk (200-239 mg/dL) does not affect all of cholesterol. Make sure you are good enough (HDL).

5. The calcium test examines the quantity of calcium not stored in your bones in your body.

For calcium levels, the typical range is 8.8-10.4 (mg/dL).

Long-term bed rest following a fractured bone, hyperparathyroidism, cancer, Paget disease and TB can produce high calcium.

Low levels of calcium might occur with low blood protein albumin, hypoparathyroidism, excessive blood phosphate concentrations, rickets and coeliac malnutrition, pancreatitis and alcoholism.

Calcium isn't only about strong bones, but it's a vital component!

6. A comprehensive urinalysis exam reveals urinary abnormalities. Lung, urinary, skin, kidney and bladder problems can all be identified by examining your pee.

All indicators of diseases which may be identified by urinalysis include high protein, the presence of crystals, pathogenic bacteria or yeast, epithelial cells, sugar, blood, acidity or pH and red or white blood cell abnormalities.

Normal urine is essentially lacking... no protein, bacteria, ketones, or glucose, and very few red or white blood cells, and crystals should be present. The typical urine pH is 6.

7. The thyroid panel shows your thyroid gland's health. It checks the TSH level in your blood and informs you whether or not your thyroid is hyperactive.

The typical range of TSH is from 0.4 to 4.0 (mIU/L).

A higher TSH level (2.0 mIU/L) suggests an active thyroid gland, causing health concerns such as weight gain, fragmented hair and nails, joint discomfort, infertility, depression and cardiac illness.

A low level of TSH suggests a thyroid gland hyperactive that generates too much thyroid hormone.

You may suffer weight loss, severe anxiety or tremors.

The difference in hypothyroid and hyperthyroid is when your levels are too high or too low. Treatments differ despite the fact that each illness is thyroid.

8. The whole blood count or CBC test examines red blood cells, white blood cells and platelets.

A normal CBC is made up of counts of white, red, platelet, hematocrit and hemoglobin.

Normal blood cell count: 3,90-5,72 trillion cells/L Normal blood cell count: 3,5-10,5 billion cells/L Normal platelet count: 150-450 trillion/L Normal hemoglobin: 12,0-17,5 grams/dL Normal hematocrit: 34,9-50,0 percent if your red blood count is low, including hemoglobin and hematocrit.

If you have the same red blood count, you may have heart problems. High red blood count causes include smoking, renal illness, heart disease, alcohol and liver disease.

A large number of white blood cells may show inflammation, infection or immunological disease.

Autoimmune diseases, cancer or bone marrow issues may produce a low white blood cell count.

The CBC is a valuable test that gives your doctor a lot of health information.

9. The 25-hydroxy vitamin D tests assess the amount of vitamin D in your body.

Vitamin D has a typical range of 20 to 40 (ng/mL).

High vitamin D may be caused by too much vitamin D and a conditions that can lead to signs of renal impairment, called hypervitaminosis D.

Low vitamin D may occur with liver and renal diseases, lack of dietary vitamin D, lack of sunshine exposure, poor absorption and usage of some medicinal products.

Most individuals suffer from a shortage of vitamin D, which is a pity as you can just get it out. Order a vitamin, mineral or dietary test 10. 10. The folate or folic acid test detects follic acid in the body; one of several forms of vitamin B.

The typical range of follic acid in the blood is between 2.7 to 17.0 (ng/mL).

More than normal follic acids are generally not harmful, but may suggest a deficit in vitamin B-12.

Lower follic acid levels may suggest anemia, malabsorption, vitamin and mineral absorption issues or a follic acid deficit.

CHAPTER 3

CONTINUATION OF HOW TO READ BLOOD TEST RESULTS

A sample of blood is generally checked with three primary tests for a daily routine check: a complete blood count (CBC) of a comprehensive metabolic panel (CMP) of a lipid panel (or profile) These tests provide several particular findings. However, many reports merely provide a single column of test results under "Test Name" rather than grouping the findings under each of the three tests. It is useful for your lab report to comprehend the link between the test results. Here are simple explanations of the three main tests and the findings mentioned most frequently.

Complete blood count (CBC) The first list under the "Test Name" column shows the CBC results, or the entire blood count, in various blood test results. The CBC measures the main blood components: red blood cells, white blood cells and platelets.

The CBC also detects the oxygen-carrying protein, hemoglobin and the ratio of red to fluid blood cells (plasma).

The results of blood tests assist your physician discover infections and allergies or diagnose possible illnesses and disorders such as anemia and leukemia.

White blood cell (WBC) count

The White blood cell count is often demonstrated to be the initial CBC test. White blood cells are a significant component of your body's immune system and are also termed leukocytes.

When you have an infection or an allergic response, your body generates more WBCs. There are five main categories of WBCs (described below), although many results of blood tests indicate them in the lower end of the CBC findings.

WBC count might potentially provide insights into your heart health. A 2018 study revealed that an elevated WBC count predicted heart disease, and notably stroke, among smokers. The report frequently shows a trusted source of red blood cells (RBCs). RBCs supply oxygen to your body's tissues.

High RBC numbers may be caused by dehydration, renal issues or heart disease. Low RBC numbers can suggest anemia, deficits in nutrition, injury to the bone marrow, or renal issues.

A high RBC might also suggest fatty liver disease which causes fat to grow and harm your liver. It might be a warning for people with obesity, type 2 diabetes, and high cholesterol because these conditions relate to fatty liver disease.Trusted

Source hemoglobin, hematocrit, and more These results are often presented under the RBC section, as they examine your red blood cell health and function.

Your doctor can aid with his measurement if your organs and tissues get adequate oxygen.

The findings of hematocrit indicate the blood volume of red blood cells. Low hematocrit may indicate anemia, loss of blood, or lack in vitamins. Dehydration or liver or heart problems might cause a surge.

Blood cells are commonly called corpuscles. The average corpuscular value measures the average red blood cell size. A deficit in vitamin B-12 or anemia may lead to aberrant RBCs.

Mean corpuscular hemoglobin quantifies the hemoglobin

average in RBCs. This is typically assessed along with the mean corpuscular hemoglobin (MCHC) concentration, which assesses the average hemoglobin percentage of RBCs.

Platelets and platelet mean value (MPV) Typically these two tests are next. Platelets are blood cell fragments. They help heal wounds and prevent excessive bleeding by generating coagulations.

A low number of platelets —
less than 150,000 platelets per
microliter (mcL) — might
suggest an excessive bleeding
risk whereas a large number
(400,000 or more) can signal a
blood clot danger.

The medium platelet value test
examines the average platelet
number. The results for the
five white blood cells,
basophiles, eosinophils,
neutrophils, lymphocytes and
monocytes, often appear under
the red blood cell results list,

can help to diagnose bleeding, bone marrow disorders and provide clues to inflammatory diseases, including cardiovascular disease, lupus, and rheumatoid arthritis.

The measurement of these cells' number and health is important in the identification of diseases and allergies.

For instance, neutrophils are like blood EMTs. They are among the first immune cells to reach the site of an infection. Basophils, another kind of immune cell, have tiny enzyme particles that release allergies and asthma.

The phrase "metabolism" in this portion of your blood work results may recall the number on the scale (and perhaps hundreds of diet books with the words "mega" and "blast" yelling all capitals).

In fact, this test group offers a far larger picture of the chemical balance and metabolism of your body.

In order to be clear, "metabolism" refers to all the physical and chemical processes in your body converting or using energy (breathing, controlling body temperature, etc.).

Electrolytes CMP offers information on electrolytes,

blood minerals that impact the quantity of water in your body, blood acidity and muscle performance. Electrolytes

CMP testing for common electrolytes include calcium, chloride, magnesium, phosphorus, potassium and sodium.

Furthermore, the CMP typically measures chemicals such as bilirubin, albumin and creatinine.

When your body breaks down hemoglobin, bilirubin develops. The bile and blood are detected, and too much might suggest jaundice.

Albumin, the primary blood plasma protein, is the clear, yellowish blood fluid containing blood cells. Low albumin levels may suggest malnutrition, inflammation and illnesses of the liver and kidneys.

Creatinine is a creatine chemical waste product that provides muscle energy. Creatine is a popular supplement as it might enable you to break down your weightlifting goals. However, because your kidneys eliminate creatinine, high amounts may indicate impaired renal function.

Fasting glucose test The fasting glucose test is frequently another component of the CMP which does not require you to eat at least 8 hours prior. Abnormal amounts of glucose might be an indication of diabetes.

Glucose is a simple sugar produced by your body from carbs, which might impact the outcome of the test.

Tip: Plan the blood work in the morning, if feasible, for the first time, to avoid "hangries" that are a legitimate problem.

At Greatist, we're not cool with a "fat speech" that is body negative. But it's completely fine to talk about your lipids (along with the fat in your body) in your blood work.

It isn't all terrible, just like the fat on your plate. Your body breaks and utilizes lipids for energy. The lipid panel is a combination of tests measuring two forms of blood fat: triglycerides and cholesterol.

Triglycerides are one of your liver's main types of fat. If you wonder what impacts your level of triglyceride, line up the typical suspects of diet: sucre, fat and alcohol.

However, the levels of triglycerides are also elevated due to thyroid or liver diseases or hereditary disorders.

Two kinds of cholesterol are present: HDL and LDL.

HDL is a lipid that transports more cholesterol from your

blood to your liver for elimination. It is commonly referred to as "good" cholesterol since it is desirable in high levels and is associated with a decreased cardiovascular risk.

LDL means 'low-density lipoprotein,' which carries cholesterol into regions of your body that require cell repair. However, it can also build up inside the arteries, which is that "bad" cholesterol is commonly termed.

The increased risk of heart and blood vessel disease, particularly coronary disease, are associated with high levels of LDL cholesterol.

Maintaining the proper balance between good and bad cholesterol and a decent amount of triglycerides is crucial for the healthy lifestyle of the heart.

A greater risk of cardiovascular disease is also associated with high triglyceride levels. And study reveals that LDL cholesterol is not the only bad guy when it comes to risk of heart disease: the ratio of triglycerides to HDL cholestersterol might be troublesome, too. If your doctor is not concerned about the outcome of the report

THE END

Printed in Great Britain
by Amazon